Hypertensive cookbook for beginners

Healthy and delicious recipes to lower your blood pressure

Sam Davis

Table of Contents:
Introduction to Hypertension and Diet

Chapter 1:Understanding hypertension
The role of diet in managing hypertension
Tips for healthy eating

Chapter 2: Breakfast Recipes

Chapter 3: Snacks and Appetizers

Chapter 4: Soups and Salads

Chapter 5: Main Dishes

Chapter 6: Sides and Accompaniments

Chapter 7: Desserts

Chapter 8: Meal Planning and Preparation

Chapter 9: Conclusion and Additional Resources

Introduction to hypertension and diet

Sophia had always been a foodie. She loved eating out and trying new foods, but her indulgent lifestyle had taken a toll on her health. She was diagnosed with hypertension, and her doctor warned her that if she didn't change her lifestyle, she was at risk of serious health problems.

Sophia was determined to get her health back on track, and she began researching how to manage hypertension through diet. She learned that a diet rich in whole grains, fruits, vegetables, and lean protein could help lower her blood pressure. She also learned that reducing her intake of sodium and saturated fats was essential for managing hypertension.

Sophia embraced this new way of eating and began cooking at home more often. She experimented with new recipes, using whole grains like quinoa and brown rice, and incorporating plenty of fresh fruits and vegetables into her meals. She also cut back on processed foods, which are often high in sodium.

Sophia's dedication paid off. After a few weeks of following her new diet, she noticed that her blood pressure had started to decrease. She continued to stick to her new eating habits, and over time, her blood pressure stabilized at a healthy level. Sophia was thrilled with the results and felt healthier than she had in years.

Sophia's experience is a testament to the power of healthy eating. By making simple changes to her diet and lifestyle, she was able to reverse hypertension and improve her overall health. Her story is an inspiration to anyone struggling with hypertension or other health problems - with the right diet and lifestyle choices, it is possible to take control of your health and live your best life.

Hypertension, also known as high blood pressure, is a chronic medical condition characterized by abnormally elevated levels of pressure in the arteries. This silent killer affects millions of people worldwide, and it is a leading risk factor for cardiovascular disease, stroke, and kidney failure. Hypertension is often referred to as the "silent killer" because it can go unnoticed for years, causing damage to the body without any symptoms. This condition can be caused by several factors, including genetic predisposition, unhealthy lifestyle choices, stress, and underlying medical conditions. Despite its prevalence and severe consequences, hypertension is often preventable and treatable with lifestyle modifications and medication. Understanding hypertension and its potential consequences is crucial to managing this condition and reducing the risk of serious health problems.

Chapter 1::

Understanding hypertension

Hypertension, also known as high blood pressure, is a medical condition characterized by abnormally high levels of pressure in the arteries. Blood pressure is the force of blood pushing against the walls of the arteries, and hypertension occurs when this pressure is consistently elevated over a period of time.

Hypertension is a common condition that affects millions of people worldwide. It is often referred to as the "silent killer" because it can go unnoticed for years, causing damage to the body without any symptoms. Over time, hypertension can damage the blood vessels, heart, and other organs, increasing the risk of serious health problems like cardiovascular disease, stroke, and kidney failure.

Several factors can contribute to the development of hypertension, including genetic predisposition, unhealthy lifestyle choices, stress, and underlying medical conditions like diabetes and kidney disease. Age, gender, and race can also increase the risk of hypertension.

The good news is that hypertension is often preventable and treatable with lifestyle modifications and medication. Simple lifestyle changes like maintaining a healthy weight, regular exercise, reducing sodium and saturated fat intake, quitting smoking, and reducing stress can all help lower blood pressure. If lifestyle modifications are not enough, medication can also be used to manage hypertension.

Regular monitoring of blood pressure is crucial for understanding hypertension and managing the condition. Blood pressure readings can be taken at home or in a doctor's office, and it is important to maintain a record of these readings to track changes over time.

In conclusion, understanding hypertension is crucial to managing the condition and reducing the risk of serious health problems. By making healthy lifestyle choices and monitoring blood pressure regularly, hypertension can be prevented, managed, and even reversed, leading to better health outcomes and a higher quality of life.

The role of diet in managing hypertension

Diet plays a crucial role in managing hypertension, also known as high blood pressure. A healthy diet can help reduce blood pressure and prevent the development of hypertension in the first place. Here are some ways that diet can help manage hypertension:

Reducing Sodium Intake: Consuming too much sodium can increase blood pressure. To manage hypertension, it is recommended to limit sodium intake to 2,300 milligrams per day or less. This can be achieved by avoiding processed foods, using spices and herbs to add flavor to meals, and cooking at home more often.

Increasing Potassium Intake: Potassium can help counteract the effects of sodium on blood pressure. A diet rich in potassium can help lower blood pressure, and it is recommended to consume 3,500 milligrams per day or more. Foods like bananas, spinach, sweet potatoes, and avocados are all excellent sources of potassium.

Eating a Diet Rich in Whole Grains, Fruits, and Vegetables: A diet that is rich in whole grains, fruits, and vegetables can help manage hypertension. These foods are rich in fiber, vitamins, and minerals that can help lower blood pressure and improve overall health.

Limiting Saturated and Trans Fats: Foods that are high in saturated and trans fats can contribute to the development of hypertension. It is recommended to limit the intake of these fats and replace them with healthier fats like monounsaturated and polyunsaturated fats found in foods like nuts, seeds, and fish.

Limiting Alcohol and Caffeine: Excessive alcohol and caffeine consumption can increase blood pressure. To manage hypertension, it is recommended to limit alcohol intake to one drink per day for women and two drinks per day for men. Caffeine intake should also be limited, especially in those who are sensitive to its effects.

In conclusion, a healthy diet can help manage hypertension by reducing sodium intake, increasing potassium intake, eating a diet rich in whole grains, fruits, and vegetables, limiting saturated and trans fats, and limiting alcohol and caffeine intake. By making these dietary changes, along with other lifestyle modifications and medication if needed, hypertension can be managed and even reversed, leading to better health outcomes and a higher quality of life.

Tips for healthy eating

Maintaining a healthy diet is essential for managing hypertension, also known as high blood pressure. Here are some tips for healthy eating that can help individuals with hypertension manage their condition:

Focus on Whole Foods: Whole foods like fruits, vegetables, whole grains, lean protein, and healthy fats should make up the majority of a hypertensive person's diet. These foods are rich in nutrients, fiber, and antioxidants that can help reduce blood pressure and improve overall health.

Reduce Sodium Intake: Hypertensive individuals should limit their sodium intake to 2,300 milligrams per day or less. To reduce sodium intake, it is recommended to avoid processed foods, read food labels, and use spices and herbs to add flavor to meals.

Increase Potassium Intake: Potassium can help counteract the effects of sodium on blood pressure. Foods like bananas, spinach, sweet potatoes, and avocados are excellent sources of potassium and should be incorporated into a hypertensive person's diet.

Choose Lean Protein: Lean protein sources like fish, poultry, beans, and legumes should be included in a hypertensive person's diet. These foods are rich in protein without the saturated fat found in red meat.

Limit Saturated and Trans Fats: Foods that are high in saturated and trans fats can contribute to the development of hypertension. It is recommended to limit the intake of these fats and replace them with healthier fats like monounsaturated and polyunsaturated fats found in foods like nuts, seeds, and fish.

Limit Alcohol and Caffeine: Excessive alcohol and caffeine consumption can increase blood pressure. Hypertensive individuals should limit alcohol intake to one drink per day for women and two drinks per day for men. Caffeine intake should also be limited, especially in those who are sensitive to its effects.

Practice Mindful Eating: Hypertensive individuals should practice mindful eating by paying attention to their hunger and fullness cues, eating slowly, and avoiding distractions like TV or smartphones during meals.

In conclusion, a healthy diet is crucial for managing hypertension. Hypertensive individuals should focus on whole foods, reduce sodium intake, increase potassium intake, choose lean protein, limit saturated and trans fats, limit alcohol and caffeine, and practice mindful eating. By making these dietary changes, along with other lifestyle modifications and medication if needed, hypertension can be managed and even reversed, leading to better health outcomes and a higher quality of life.

Chapter 2:

Breakfast Recipes

For hypertensive people, it is important to follow a healthy diet to help manage their condition. A healthy breakfast is a great way to start the day and can help maintain blood pressure levels. Here are some breakfast recipe ideas for hypertensive people:

Greek Yogurt Parfait: Layer Greek yogurt, berries, and a sprinkle of granola or nuts in a parfait glass. Greek yogurt is high in protein and low in fat, making it a great breakfast option for hypertensive people. Berries are a good source of fiber and antioxidants, while granola or nuts add a satisfying crunch.

Veggie Omelet: Whisk together eggs, salt, and pepper, then pour the mixture into a non-stick skillet. Add sautéed veggies such as bell peppers, onions, and spinach to one side of the omelet and fold the other side over to enclose the veggies. Vegetables are rich in potassium and low in sodium, which is beneficial for hypertension.

Whole Grain Toast with Avocado: Toast a slice of whole-grain bread and top it with mashed avocado and a sprinkle of red pepper flakes. Avocado is high in monounsaturated fats, which can help lower blood pressure. Whole grain bread is a good source of fiber, which can also help regulate blood pressure.

Smoothie Bowl: Blend together frozen berries, spinach, almond milk, and a banana, then pour the mixture into a bowl and top it with sliced almonds and chia seeds. This smoothie bowl is packed with antioxidants and fiber, which are beneficial for hypertensive people.

Overnight Oats: Combine rolled oats, chia seeds, almond milk, and honey in a mason jar and let it sit in the refrigerator overnight. In the morning, top it with sliced bananas and a sprinkle of cinnamon. This breakfast option is rich in fiber and protein, which can help regulate blood pressure levels.

It's important to note that hypertensive people should also limit their intake of salt and processed foods. A diet rich in whole grains, fruits, vegetables, lean proteins, and low-fat dairy products is recommended for managing hypertension.

Chapter 3:

Snacks and Appetizers

Hypertension, or high blood pressure, is a common health condition that affects millions of people around the world. If you have hypertension, it's important to manage your diet to help control your blood pressure. Snacks and appetizers can be a challenge for people with hypertension because many common options are high in sodium, which can raise blood pressure. However, there are still plenty of tasty and healthy options available. Here are some snacks and appetizers that are suitable for hypertensive people:

Fresh veggies and dip: Raw vegetables like carrot sticks, cucumber slices, and cherry tomatoes are low in sodium and high in fiber, which can help lower blood pressure. Dip them in a low-sodium hummus or tzatziki sauce for added flavor.

Fresh fruit: Fruits such as apples, pears, berries, and oranges are naturally low in sodium and high in potassium, which can help lower blood pressure. Try pairing fruit with a low-fat cheese or nut butter for added protein.

Roasted nuts: Nuts like almonds, cashews, and pistachios are high in heart-healthy fats and protein. Opt for unsalted or low-sodium roasted nuts, as many store-bought varieties are loaded with salt.

Popcorn: Air-popped popcorn is a low-sodium and high-fiber snack that can help you feel full. Sprinkle it with a small amount of salt-free seasoning or nutritional yeast for added flavor.

Guacamole and veggies: Guacamole is high in healthy fats and fiber, and can be a great dip for raw veggies like celery, bell peppers, and carrots.

Deviled eggs: Hard-boiled eggs are a great source of protein and can be made into a low-sodium appetizer by using a low-sodium mustard and mayonnaise.

Edamame: Boiled edamame is a tasty and low-sodium snack that is also high in protein and fiber. Try seasoning it with a sprinkle of sesame oil and a pinch of sea salt for added flavor.

Remember to read food labels when buying snacks and appetizers and choose products that are low in sodium. Also, it's important to practice portion control, even with healthy snacks. Snacks can quickly add up in calories and sodium if you eat too much, so stick to reasonable serving sizes. By choosing healthy and low-sodium snacks, you can help manage your blood pressure and maintain a healthy diet.

Chapter 4:

Soups and Salads

Hypertension, or high blood pressure, is a medical condition that affects a significant number of people worldwide. Diet plays a crucial role in managing hypertension, and soups and salads can be excellent additions to a hypertensive person's meal plan. Here are some tips and ideas for soups and salads for hypertensive people:

Watch the Sodium Content: Sodium is a significant contributor to hypertension. When preparing soups and salads, it's important to limit the amount of sodium used. Opt for low-sodium broth, and use fresh herbs and spices to enhance the flavor instead of salt. Read labels when choosing canned ingredients, such as beans or tomatoes, to ensure they are low in sodium.

Increase Potassium: Potassium can help to counteract the effects of sodium and reduce blood pressure. Add potassium-rich ingredients to your salads and soups, such as spinach, sweet potatoes, avocados, bananas, and tomatoes.

Incorporate Healthy Fats: Healthy fats, such as those found in olive oil, nuts, and seeds, can help to lower blood pressure. Use olive oil and vinegar as a dressing for your salad, and add nuts or seeds for crunch.

Choose Lean Protein: Protein is an essential part of a balanced diet, but it's important to choose lean options to manage hypertension. Chicken, fish, and turkey are excellent choices for soups and salads. Avoid processed meats, such as bacon or sausage, which are high in sodium.

Try Different Types of Soups: Soups can be a satisfying and healthy meal option for hypertensive people. Opt for broths or vegetable-based soups, which tend to be lower in sodium than cream-based soups. Try adding lentils or beans to your soup for added protein and fiber.

Mix Up Your Salad Ingredients: Salads can be a great way to incorporate a variety of healthy ingredients into your diet. Mix up your salad ingredients to keep things interesting. Try adding fruits, such as strawberries or oranges, or vegetables, such as broccoli or bell peppers. Use a variety of greens, such as spinach, kale, or arugula, for added nutrition.

Be Mindful of Portion Sizes: While soups and salads can be healthy meal options, it's important to be mindful of portion sizes. Overeating can contribute to high blood pressure, so be sure to stick to recommended serving sizes.

In conclusion, soups and salads can be excellent meal options for hypertensive people. By choosing low-sodium ingredients, incorporating potassium-rich foods, and adding healthy fats and lean protein, you can create satisfying and nutritious meals that help to manage hypertension.

Chapter 5:

Main Dishes

Hypertension, or high blood pressure, is a common health condition that affects so many people worldwide. Diet plays a crucial role in managing hypertension, and consuming a balanced and healthy diet is crucial to prevent complications associated with high blood pressure. Here are some main dishes that hypertensive people can enjoy as part of a healthy diet:

Grilled chicken or fish: Grilled chicken or fish is a great source of lean protein and is low in fat. Season with herbs and spices, such as rosemary or black pepper, for added flavor without the need for salt.

Brown rice and vegetable stir-fry: Brown rice is a complex carbohydrate that can help regulate blood sugar levels and reduce blood pressure. A vegetable stir-fry made with colorful vegetables, such as bell peppers, carrots, and broccoli, can add fiber, vitamins, and minerals to the dish.

Baked sweet potato and salmon: Sweet potatoes are a rich source of potassium, which can help regulate blood pressure. Baked salmon is a great source of omega-3 fatty acids, which can help reduce inflammation and lower blood pressure.

Lentil soup: Lentils are a good source of protein and fiber and can help regulate blood sugar levels. A lentil soup made with low-sodium vegetable broth, vegetables, and herbs can be a filling and nutritious main dish.

Quinoa salad: Quinoa is a complete protein that can help lower blood pressure and reduce inflammation. A quinoa salad made with colorful vegetables, such as cherry tomatoes, cucumbers, and bell peppers, can add fiber and antioxidants to the dish.

Turkey chili: Ground turkey is a lean source of protein that can be used to make a delicious and healthy chili. Use low-sodium canned beans, diced tomatoes, and chili powder for added flavor without the need for salt.

When preparing main dishes for hypertensive people, it is essential to limit the use of salt and opt for herbs and spices instead. Additionally, avoid using processed and high-sodium ingredients, such as canned soups and sauces, and opt for fresh ingredients whenever possible.

Chapter 6:

Sides and Accompaniments

Hypertension, or high blood pressure, affects millions of people worldwide and diet plays a crucial role in managing this condition. Consuming a balanced and healthy diet that includes sides and accompaniments with low sodium content is essential for hypertensive people. Here are some healthy and delicious sides and accompaniments for hypertensive people:

Roasted vegetables: Roasting vegetables with a little bit of olive oil, black pepper, and herbs can add flavor without the need for salt. Colorful vegetables, such as sweet potatoes, carrots, and bell peppers, can provide fiber, vitamins, and minerals.

Steamed broccoli: Steaming broccoli until it is tender can be a healthy and delicious side dish. Broccoli is a great source of vitamins and minerals, including vitamin C and potassium.

Brown rice: Brown rice is a complex carbohydrate that can help regulate blood sugar levels and reduce blood pressure. It can be served as a side dish or used as a base for a grain bowl.

Quinoa: Quinoa is a complete protein that can help lower blood pressure and reduce inflammation. It can be served as a side dish or used as a base for a salad.

Hummus: Hummus is a tasty and healthy dip made from chickpeas and olive oil. It can be served with fresh vegetables, such as carrot sticks, celery, and cucumber slices, for a healthy and low-sodium snack.

Guacamole: Guacamole is a dip made from avocado, lime juice, and cilantro. It is a great source of healthy fats and can be served with fresh vegetables or whole-grain crackers.

Salsa: Salsa is a low-sodium dip made from tomatoes, onions, and peppers. It can be served with baked tortilla chips or fresh vegetables for a healthy and flavorful snack.

When preparing sides and accompaniments for hypertensive people, it is essential to limit the use of salt and opt for herbs and spices instead. Additionally, avoid using processed and high-sodium ingredients, such as canned beans and sauces, and opt for fresh ingredients whenever possible.

Chapter 7:

Desserts

Diet plays a crucial role in managing hypertension, or high blood pressure. Hypertensive people need to be careful with their sugar intake, as excessive sugar consumption can increase blood pressure levels. However, that does not mean they cannot enjoy a sweet treat now and then. Here are some healthy dessert options for hypertensive people:

Fresh fruit: Fresh fruit is a great way to satisfy a sweet craving without the need for added sugar. Choose fruits that are low in sugar, such as berries, melons, and citrus fruits.

Dark chocolate: Dark chocolate is said to be rich in antioxidants which helps to lower blood pressure. Choose a high-quality dark chocolate with at least 70% cocoa content.

Greek yogurt with berries: Greek yogurt is a great source of protein and can be combined with fresh berries for a healthy and delicious dessert. Add a drizzle of honey for added sweetness if needed.

Baked apples: Baked apples are a great low-sugar dessert option. Simply core an apple and fill it with a mixture of cinnamon, nuts, and honey. Bake until tender and serve with a dollop of Greek yogurt.

Chia seed pudding: Chia seed pudding is a healthy and satisfying dessert option. Combine chia seeds with almond milk and sweetener of choice, such as honey or maple syrup, and refrigerate until the mixture thickens. Top with fresh fruit and nuts for added flavor and texture.

Banana ice cream: Banana ice cream is a healthy and delicious alternative to traditional ice cream. Simply freeze ripe bananas and blend them in a food processor until smooth and creamy. Add cocoa powder or peanut butter for added flavor.

When preparing desserts for hypertensive people, it is essential to limit the use of sugar and opt for natural sweeteners, such as honey or maple syrup, instead. Additionally, avoid using processed and high-sugar ingredients, such as refined sugar and white flour, and opt for whole food ingredients whenever possible.

Chapter 8:

Meal Planning and Preparation

Hypertension, commonly known as high blood pressure, is a condition that affects millions of people around the world. It is characterized by the pressure of blood against the walls of arteries being consistently high, which can lead to various health problems. Meal planning and preparation are important considerations for hypertensive people, as a healthy diet can help to manage blood pressure levels and reduce the risk of complications.

Here are some tips for meal planning and preparation for hypertensive people:

Limit sodium intake: Sodium, which is found in salt and processed foods, can raise blood pressure levels. It is important to limit sodium intake to less than 2,300 milligrams per day, and ideally less than 1,500 milligrams per day for those with hypertension. Try to cook with fresh herbs and spices instead of salt, and avoid processed foods that are high in sodium.

Increase potassium intake: Potassium can help to counteract the effects of sodium and lower blood pressure levels. Good sources of potassium include fruits such as bananas, avocados, and oranges, as well as vegetables such as spinach, sweet potatoes, and tomatoes.

Choose lean protein: Protein is an important part of a healthy diet, but some sources of protein, such as red meat, can be high in saturated fat, which can raise blood pressure levels. Choose lean sources of protein such as chicken, fish, beans, and tofu.

Include whole grains: Whole grains are a good source of fiber, which can help to lower blood pressure levels. Choose whole grain bread, pasta, and rice instead of refined grains.

Incorporate fruits and vegetables: Fruits and vegetables are low in sodium and high in potassium, fiber, and other nutrients that can help to lower blood pressure levels. Aim to include a variety of fruits and vegetables in your diet.

Plan ahead: Planning ahead can make it easier to stick to a healthy diet. Plan your meals for the week and make a grocery list to ensure that you have healthy ingredients on hand. Consider meal prepping to make it easier to eat healthy meals throughout the week.

Cook at home: Cooking at home can help you to control the amount of sodium and other unhealthy ingredients in your meals. Try to cook meals from scratch instead of relying on processed foods or eating out.

In summary, meal planning and preparation are important considerations for hypertensive people. A healthy diet that is low in sodium, high in potassium, and includes lean protein, whole grains, fruits, and vegetables can help to manage blood pressure levels and reduce the risk of complications. Planning ahead and cooking at home can also make it easier to stick to a healthy diet.

Chapter 9:

Conclusion and Additional Resources

Incorporating healthy and delicious recipes into your diet can have a significant impact on reducing your blood pressure levels. By choosing foods that are low in sodium, high in potassium, and rich in nutrients, you can improve your overall health and well-being.

It's important to remember that diet alone may not be enough to lower your blood pressure. It's also essential to engage in regular exercise, maintain a healthy weight, reduce stress, and limit alcohol consumption. A holistic approach to managing blood pressure is necessary for optimal health outcomes.

In conclusion, by making small dietary changes and incorporating these healthy and delicious recipes into your routine, you can take control of your blood pressure and improve your overall health.

Additional Resources:

The American Heart Association:
https://www.heart.org/
The National Heart, Lung, and Blood Institute:
https://www.nhlbi.nih.gov/
Dietary Approaches to Stop Hypertension
(DASH) Diet:
https://www.nhlbi.nih.gov/health-topics/dash-eating-plan
Centers for Disease Control and Prevention:
https://www.cdc.gov/bloodpressure/index.htm